FAT BOB
How to Lose We:
Your Blood Pressure

"If a 220 lbs pizza munching, lager swilling
Glaswegian can do it – so can you!"

About the author

Bobby Livingston is FAT BOB SLIM.

He is the originator of the FAT BOB SLIM regime. He is also a reformed pizza munching, lager swilling Glaswegian.

At the beginning of 2014 he weighed 220 lbs and was on the cusp of being classified as clinically obese.

Unbeknown to him at the age of 50 he had developed high blood pressure and was sleepwalking his way to illness and an early grave.

After experiencing the shock of his life at his local doctor's surgery he decided it was time to act, time to lose weight.

FAT BOB SLIM is his personal story and regime, one that has enabled him to shed the pounds and slash his blood pressure.

As FAT BOB SLIM says:

"If a 220 lbs pizza munching, lager swilling Glaswegian can do it – so can you!"

When not evangelizing about healthy eating, walking and weight loss, FAT BOB SLIM passes his time as a writer and professional speaker.

He lives in Glasgow, Scotland with his wife and son.

FAT BOB SLIM: How to Lose Weight & Slash Your Blood Pressure

Bobby Livingston

Published by The Change Agents (Publishing)
Glasgow G43 1JY, Scotland
admin@thechangeagents.co.uk

First published 2014

This book is not a medical guide and should not be relied upon as such. Please consult a qualified medical practitioner before beginning any exercise, fasting or diet modification. The publisher and author are not responsible for any specific or underlying health needs that require medical supervision.

For details of paperback bulk purchase discounts contact
admin@thechangeagents.co.uk

A CIP catalogue record for this book is available from the British Library.

ISBN: 978-0-9571054-5-4

Cover by Laura Fergus Design
Photographer: Vin Mcguire

Every effort has been made to contact copyright holders. However, the publisher will be glad to rectify in future editions any inadvertent omissions brought to its attention.

A personal note from
FAT BOB SLIM

Are you overweight?

At the beginning of 2014 I was a 220 lbs pizza munching, lager swilling Glaswegian on the cusp of obesity.

I was fat, getting fatter, and I knew it. But I had done nothing about it.

Does that sound familiar to you?

What I didn't know, until an unrelated visit to my doctor, was I had developed dangerously high blood pressure.

High blood pressure is known as the "silent killer." It significantly increases the risk of developing heart disease and having a stroke amongst a range of other nasties that can lead to an early grave.

As the father of a son who is my world I simply had to get my act together. I had to be about for him: I had to be about to see him grow up, I had to be about to guide him through school, to experience his cheekiness, and to hear his hyena-like laughter...

Is your motivation to lose weight similar?

Today, just four months on, I have shed over 40 lbs. I am also slim and my blood pressure is normal.

How I transformed myself from a pizza munching, lager swilling Glaswegian into a slim, active, vegetable eater is revealed through FAT BOB SLIM.

My hope is that through my words I will inspire you to lose weight and slash your blood pressure too.

I want to motivate you to transform your life, regain your health, and to live longer. And nothing will give me greater satisfaction than to hear from you to that effect.

In the interim...

What I have written here for you is simple yet practical.

More importantly, it works.

Believe me, it works!

I have listened to what the leading doctors and health experts around the world advise and brought together four key components that I know make a difference.

These are: diet modification, fasting, walking and stress relief.

FAT BOB SLIM is thus a life transformation.

It is not just a book about dieting.

Personally, I hate the thought of dieting.

Instead, for you I have made weight loss and blood pressure reduction easy to understand and easy to achieve.

So easy in fact that:

"If a 220 lbs pizza munching, lager swilling Glaswegian can do it – so can you!"

All it takes is a little commitment.

All it takes is for you to care enough.

My friend, your health is important.

Make it your top priority.

And whatever you do, don't die of ignorance.

Read FAT BOB SLIM with an open mind. Follow what it tells you and let the magic of weight loss and blood pressure reduction begin...

Bobby Livingston (aka FAT BOB SLIM)
6th June 2014
Glasgow, Scotland.

Contents

The shock of my life...

Aging happens.

So does gaining weight.

Additional pounds crept up on me, slowly, so slowly I didn't care enough to notice it happening.

But it happened.

Then in 2013 I attended a pre-Christmas get together with the family; much pizza, alcohol and ice cream were consumed, mainly by me. Essential photographs for the family album were taken.

Next day I saw them posted on Facebook. They looked great. But one, in particular, troubled me. I looked and saw a fat guy and thought surely that isn't me.

But you know what?

It was.

It was a shock to the system.

But not half the shock that was soon to follow in the doctor's surgery. More of this in a second...

How did this happen to me?

The guy that used to run 3 times each week had now become a FAT BOB.

I'd known it all along really. My trousers were getting tighter, I was buying bigger waist sizes, larger belts with more notches, my belly was looking rotund, a bit like Santa Claus, and I was having difficulty bending to tie my shoe laces. I also had a persistent backache I put down to bad posture. I'd packed in my running and fitness regime too due to a knee problem. McDonald's was becoming my regular haunt; the drive-through team virtually had my meal prepared just by number plate recognition alone - seriously!

Then, with an annoying, recurring inner ear condition, I attended my local doctor. In the course of events he took my blood pressure reading. The reading wasn't high; it was super high. In fact, at that time it was comfortably in the stage 2 hypertension range and rising.

That is about as bad as it gets.

That second shock to my system was a hammer blow.

I knew I had to act. I had put my health at risk.

That was unforgivable.

After I got home I began to read about hypertension and being overweight. What I read wasn't pretty:

common concerns included the potential for a heart attack or a stroke. My next door neighbour had had a stroke not long ago. She could hardly speak, one side of her face was frozen, and her thinking was still a bit fuzzy. I didn't fancy that. Not in a million years, well a human lifetime anyway.

Then there was the increased risk of developing cancer and the fact my kidneys would be struggling.

I sank in despair.

To rub salt in to my wounds the health websites I looked at mentioned diabetes and erectile dysfunction too.

Heavens!

I wanted to be a fully functioning man not an invalid.

Panic set in, my blood pressure soared in response and my ears rang like church bells.

I simply had to act.

But although my doctor had said "don't worry" I was doing the opposite. He also said "try losing some weight." That was fine but I wasn't sure where or how to start.

I'd never dieted before.

I Googled diets and was presented with hundreds, if not thousands, of options: Atkins, Paleo, Mediterranean, Pineapple, Weight Watchers, DASH, Ornish, etc...

So there I was, this well-educated guy with an honours degree in science, struggling to make any sense of what I saw before me.

Do I go down this route or that route?

What to do for the best?

Dilemma.

I was beginning to realise why so many people simply give up dieting and go back to their regular pattern of eating.

Choosing a diet is just too confusing.

Then by chance I saw a book on the Amazon website for the Fast Diet by Dr Michael Mosley & Mimi Spencer.

Funnily, I had watched Dr Mosley's BBC2 Horizon programme: Eat, Fast and Live Longer during the summer.

The book was his follow-up to the programme.

The health benefits associated with fasting are many: losing weight and reducing blood pressure are just two.

Better still the Fast Diet is what is known as a 5:2 diet: 5 days of the week you eat normally; 2 days you significantly reduce your calorie intake – 500 for women and 600 for men.

At first glance that sounded doable to me.

So it isn't really fasting as I understand it but instead it is all about being able to go for a long spell during a fast day without eating; and when you do eat you consume protein and lots of healthy vegetables but not carbohydrate.

Dr Mosley says that fasting "lowers the risk of a range of diseases, including diabetes, heart disease and cancer."[i] He also points out the pounds will fly off.

I ordered the book without hesitation.

It is a great read and highly recommended. Through his book Dr Mosley convinced me of the combined health and weight loss benefits that would follow through intermittent fasting.

I thought I'd experiment and give it a go.

But fasting for 2 days of the week, as powerful as it is, is not the Holy Grail. I needed to eat less in general on the other 5 days of the week and exercise too.

The Herald newspaper's editorial headline "An urgent exercise in dealing with obesity,"[ii] made interesting reading. Steven Blair, an American professor of public health noted that Scotland was in danger of sleepwalking into obesity. According to official statistics more than one quarter of my fellow countrymen and women are already obese. That is not far behind America. Scotland and America: the land of the free; the land of the fat.

Professor Blair says we must change our thinking from 'I must go on a diet' to 'I must become more active'. In the same article, Sir Harry Burns, Scotland's chief medical officer, warned that a lack of exercise is as damaging to our health as smoking, alcohol abuse and diabetes combined.

That is simply staggering.

Those statements from health and medical experts knocked me sideways, literally.

It wasn't just a diet I needed but a life transformation.

Luckily, I have always been a keen walker so I dusted down my old walking boots. Daily walking it would be from now on. This was an easy win. I was playing to my strengths.

My thinking was very much one step at a time; one small step to help turn the tide. In truth I felt as if I was clutching at straws. But at least I was clutching at something. Hope is a great thing. But, as I have found out, acting when you have hope in your heart is even greater. It can literally move mountains; shed pounds and slash your blood pressure.

At this time I decided to invest in some equipment: an Omron blood pressure monitor, a set of Salter scales, and a Beurer heart rate monitor for my walking.

The old statistician in me came to life and I began to log all the daily data on an Excel spreadsheet. I charted my weight, body fat, body water, systolic and diastolic blood pressure, and my heart rate. I collated moving averages in the hope of observing positive trends.

Put simply I was taking control, taking steps to get my health back to how it should be.

Then in my daily blood pressure measurements I began to notice spikes. These occurred after stress.

These spikes also happened when I had food that was high in salt.

Online investigation led me to the DASH diet (Dietary Approaches to Stop Hypertension). It also led me to understand and then begin to practise yoga breathing exercises to induce a sense of calmness and contentment in my life.

FAT BOB SLIM is thus not really a diet but my new way of living and is a combination of fasting, diet modification, exercise, and stress management. These four elements together have proven to be supremely powerful allies in my battle to regain health.

I've had my ups and downs on this journey but this I know to be true: I've not just started a fad but instead initiated a deeply meaningful and personal life transformation.

I call it the FAT BOB SLIM programme.

It is my personal life changing regime.

And the best thing is you can do it too.

Just substitute your name for BOB in FAT BOB SLIM and get started...

Today, as I write this for you, I have lost over 40 lbs. My average systolic blood pressure has fallen by 39% and my diastolic by 26%. And I am within my ideal BMI (Body Mass Index) weight range with the downward trend continuing in a managed way.

I have cut my weight and slashed my blood pressure.

My health risks are reducing day by day.

It is not too far-fetched to say I might just have saved my life.

If you are carrying some extra weight the time to act is NOW.

My wife says the benefits of FAT BOB SLIM are so noticeable you should have started yesterday...

So what are you waiting for?

Be brave.

Take the first step right now.

Come, join me and I'll take you through my personal journey; I'll explain what I did, why I did what I did, and the resultant effect on my weight and blood pressure.

Start my FAT BOB SLIM regime today and you'll learn about fasting, diet modification, exercise and stress management.

FAT BOB SLIM saved my life.

It might just save your life too.

Happy reading!

And good luck on your FAT BOB SLIM journey.

Dump the junk food

Everywhere I go I am surrounded by junk food.

The supermarket shelves are full of it: crisps (chips and dips for my American friends), fizzy, sugar-laden soft drinks, cakes and pastries, biscuits (cookies), snack bars, confectionery...

Are you drooling at the thought of it all?

Then add in some processed packaged foods and microwave meals.

Add alcohol into the mix too.

And let's not forget the visits to McDonald's and KFC and Pizza Hut. Not bad in moderation but what if it eating there has become a regular habit?

Oh and in Scotland: fish and chips. Who can resist a good fry up: the smell of pickled onion, the crispy batter, and the salt and vinegar combo. Or if you are from Edinburgh: the salt and sauce combo.

"Lovely jubbly" as Del Boy would have said in Only Fools and Horses.

Even in most offices the vending machines are full of junk food: coffee with sugar, lemon tea with sugar, syrupy colas, chocolate bars... Just what the average sedentary office worker needs to pass the time until 5pm!

And sadly we are easily hoodwinked by the marketing boys and girls where food is concerned: many of the supposedly healthy fruit juice drinks have such high sugar content the medical profession are calling for them to be removed from the list of 5-a-day.

Go to your local sports centre and you can fuel-up on sugary drinks too. Why not do it after a work-out and totally defeat any benefit you may have accrued.

A vicious cycle is it not?

I love the cinema. I love taking my son to see the films I wouldn't go to see myself as an adult. But even there we are not safe: popcorn: salt or sweet? Fizzy drinks: full sugar, diet or Max option? But diet and Max contain aspartame sweetener and the jury is out with regard to whether it has the same effect on the body's insulin levels as sugar does.[iii] The only difference for sure is aspartame has next to no calories, and that is surely a false compromise, if ever there was one, on the diabetes front.

At school my son buys chocolate bars and stuffs his blazer pockets with the wrappers. For some reason he seems to think I won't notice his indulgences. Too bad son, you've been caught Hershey-handed!

In the main shopping street there are take-away outlets everywhere. They have filled the gaps left by retailers moving to out of town shopping centres. Take-away, bank, charity shop, confectioners, pub, another bank just in case you need some more money to spend at the next take-away or pub or bakers.

And so it goes on.

Go to the out of town shopping centres and the weary shopper is offered a selection of Baskin Robbins' ice creams and Dunkin' Donuts' doughnuts, or a personal favourite of a Starbucks' latte with a cinnamon swirl.

And if all this late night shopping is too much why not pop into the Burger King next to the motorway for your evening meal?

Seriously: junk food is everywhere.

When I log into Facebook I get adverts for Kit-Kat chocolate fingered biscuits.

When I am browsing websites Google reminds me to buy some pizza. My letter box reminds me too with flyer after flyer for the local Papa John's pizza take-away, Indian or Chinese...

When I switch the TV on to sit back and relax of an evening I am bombarded with adverts for junk food:

Domino Pizza, Coca-Cola, Subway, Pepsi, McDonald's, Irn Bru...

It goes on and on 24/7 thanks to digital TV, the internet and mobile technology.

Every corner of my life is encroached upon by junk food.

Yet, it is usually high in sugar, saturated fats and salt.

Take too much of any of these and you put your health at risk.

That is a fact.

And the outcome: rising obesity levels, a diabetes epidemic, high blood pressure with increased risk of heart attack, stroke and cancer too. Not pleasant.

That should be enough for anyone to stop and re-evaluate but, if I am honest, I knew that and did nothing about it. I required a shock to my system to really startle me and make me want to take positive action.

Thank God for a troublesome inner ear condition or I may never have visited my doctor. Thank God my doctor was wise enough to take my blood pressure reading.

Thank you God. I owe you one...

The first thing I did was thus to dump the junk food.

It is easy to do.

And if you are serious about wanting to lose weight and slash your blood pressure you have to do it too.

Dump the junk food.

Dump the bags of crisps, pastries and biscuits.

Dump the pizzas, burgers and fried food too.

Dump the alcohol.

For me it was time to get back to basics with healthy fruits and vegetables, lean meats, oily fish, porridge and wholemeal bread. Funnily enough, the sort of food my dear old mother used to make when I was a child. In those halcyon days nothing came out of a packet. It was bought fresh on the day, prepared by my mother's fine hands and lovingly cooked and served before me.

I had to get back to that.

In truth it was easier to do than I believed.

Seriously, if you want to lose weight and slash your blood pressure you need to do it too.

No ifs, no buts.

As the Nike advert says: JUST DO IT!

I promise you this: you will never regret the day you dumped the junk food.

It was a significant turning point for me; it will be a significant turning point for you too.

Have I been tempted since my decision? Hell, yes! Have I consumed any junk food whilst on FAT BOB SLIM? Hell yes, but only very, very occasionally. And that is the way it should be; a treat, not an everyday or every week expectation.

And in any case once you learn to fast you re-educate your stomach and taste buds. The one thing you will want more of is good, healthy food not stodge. Your body will want it light.

Get your focus right from the outset.

Healthy foods are the way forward. I am convinced vegetables are heaven sent. They are full of natural goodness and health inducing properties. Why I had ignored them is part of my West of Scotland cultural heritage which I will tell you more about in the following chapter.

In the meantime, take my advice, get cracking: dump the junk food.

Learn to love your vegetables

Do you love your vegetables?

Do you pack your plate full of them?

Do you have more vegetables on a plate than you do of fish or meat when you sit down for dinner?

Do you?

I'll come back to this in a second...

I grew up in Glasgow, the biggest city in Scotland.

The city has a huge industrial, heavy engineering and ship building past. The river Clyde, which flows through the city, has launched thousands of ships including the world famous RMS Lusitania, RMS Queen Mary, and SS Queen Elizabeth.

These were special ships, beautiful, elegant, world class.

The term Clydebuilt was synonymous with excellence is design, engineering and craftsmanship.

It is ironic that the passengers who cruised on these magnificent feats of engineering dined far more extravagantly than the men who laboured so hard to create them.

Blood, sweat and tears went into every rivet that launched these ships on the Clyde.

Glasgow was then a rich and booming city: throughout the 19th and early 20th centuries it was referred to in awe as the second city of the British Empire.

Cue song from local boys Hue and Cry:

> "In the second city of the Empire,
> Mother Glasgow watches all her weans,
> Trying hard to feed her little starlings..."iv

She was trying hard then and she is trying hard still to feed all of her inhabitants.

Not that long ago, the fumes from the industrial chimneys and steam engines would cover the city in smog, ash and dirt.

My dear old mother would scream when I was a baby. Not because I was driving her crazy but rather that a steam train had stopped at the local signal and blown sooty, black ash all over her painstakingly hand washed sheets which were drying on the line in the back garden.

It was a city of smog and industrial pollution. It offered enormous wealth for the few but grinding poverty for the many who laboured at the sharp end. And with poverty came a culture of not eating vegetables and fruit. Heavens, some fruits weren't even known about in Scotland until after the Second World War.

I once saw an old TV clip that showed a young boy being given a banana to eat, he tried it with the skin on, bit into the horrible yellow stringy covering – he simply didn't know any better. We were playing catch-up with fruit and vegetables back then and we are still playing catch-up in many quarters of our great city: a city, where male life expectancy, in some parts, is as low as 54 years. Let me just say that again: male life expectancy in some parts of Glasgow, my home city, is just 54 years.

Yes, in the Calton district of Glasgow men live on average to a ripe old age of just 53.9 years old. Life expectancy for a man in Iraq, despite the bombs and horrors of conflict, is 67 years.[v]

Something is terribly wrong.

The prevalent culture is that eating vegetables is for wimps. The mind-set is that real men don't eat veg. The NHS still struggles to get its 5 portions of fruit and vegetables a day message across to the masses. And it breaks my heart.

Popeye ate spinach for the iron and the strength it gave him but my fellow Glaswegians turned to Irn Bru, a sugary drink, to put some oomph in their pencil.

Irn Bru is considered by many Glaswegians to have mystical healing properties, particularly where a hang-over is concerned. Even today you will see young, and not so young, men walking the city's streets early on a morning clutching a bottle of Irn Bru under their arm. They have a look on their face as if they have just been to the pharmacist and exited with a secret cure-all, an elixir for life and the human condition, something only owners of a bottle of the ginger coloured, bubble gum flavoured Irn Bru are privy to.

I once took a good friend of mine to Café Jean Claude on the South Side of Glasgow. That evening Jean Claude served a beautiful Alsace menu. I swear that I looked on in astonishment as every single piece of vegetable was put to the side of his plate, only the meat was eaten. My friend was from Clydebank. He lived in the shadow of the great ship building yard that launched the QE2. On the way home he proclaimed he was hungry, walked into the local fish and chip shop and bought a bag of fried onion rings and proceeded to devour them.

Alsace cuisine 0: Fried onion rings 1.

Years have passed since the great Cunard ships were launched from Clydebank; years have passed since Glasgow was the 2nd City of the Empire, but the prevalent culture of not eating vegetables remains.

It is deeply saddening.

But friend I want to talk to you today like an evangelist would.

I want to talk from the bottom of my heart.

I want to talk to you as a convert.

I want to talk to you as a born again vegetable eater.

Vegetables are good.

Vegetables are your friends.

Vegetables have magical qualities.

They will heal you and rejuvenate you.

Vegetables will bring you lasting good health and happiness.

Real men do eat vegetables; in fact, without them real men die young.

If you really want to change your life for the better, if you really desire to lose weight and slash your blood pressure, then believe me that vegetables are your friend.

Real men eat vegetables because they know how wonderful they are.

Real men eat vegetables and are not afraid to proclaim to their fellow citizens that they do so.

They are proud of the fact.

They are proud to eat cabbage, cauliflower, courgette and cucumber.

They are proud to eat beetroot, beans and broccoli.

They are proud to eat potatoes, peas and parsnips.

And when summer comes they are proud to mix some leaves of lettuce with vine tomatoes, chopped red onion, yellow peppers, and pitted olives. They are proud to pour on some extra virgin olive oil and to garnish with a covering of finely chopped parsley and a drizzle of lemon juice.

They are proud because they know how good it is for them.

They are proud because every mouthful is a fight against disease and an early death.

They are proud because they are at the forefront of a new trend, a new trend that will set the bar high for the generations yet to come.

They are proud that their children will inherit a new way of eating.

They are proud of what they have done.

They are proud because, despite how difficult it may seem, eating vegetables is easy, it is tasty and it's fun.

Learn to make vegetables your friends.

Seriously, they are packed with goodness.

Forget the sugary drinks, the alcohol and fried food.

Make every plate you eat at dinner time have far more vegetables on it than you do of fish or meat.

Make that your goal from now on and you'll see the weight drop off and your blood pressure begin to reduce.

Vegetables are your friends.

Now, some important details:

Are you sitting comfortably? Then I'll begin...

Did you know that a beetroot contains chemicals that protect against coronary heart disease and stroke? Better than that, the wee red coloured beetroot bulb lowers your cholesterol levels and has anti-aging effects too.[vi]

I'm not saying you are going to be the next Cliff Richard but it is worth a go isn't it?

Now, be honest with me, have you eaten a beetroot lately?

Why not?

It is doing you a favour; it is your friend.

Or do you keep your friends at arm's length and only visit them once in a blue moon?

Did you know that broccoli contains chemicals that help protect against prostate cancer? Yup, that green stalk is God's special health agent here on earth. Pop into your local supermarket or grocer and say hello to him. Say "Hello broccoli, how are you pal?" And, just in case you didn't know, it protects against the risk of developing colon, bladder, pancreatic and breast cancers too.[vii]

Seriously, you want to be friendly with these guys. They might look green and simple, they might not talk back to you when you speak to them but they pack one hell of a punch in your body's defence against disease and aging.

Learn to make them your friends.

Now, let me ask you, have you eaten some asparagus lately?

I recall as a child going for a day out with the church and having an evening meal where asparagus soup was served. I'd never heard of it. This wee kid from

Glasgow was none the wiser when a plate with lime coloured contents was put down in front of him but I tried it anyway: it was tasty, very tasty. And the moral of this: get your kids started young where vegetables are concerned.

Did you know asparagus is a good source of calcium and potassium?[viii]

Calcium maintains healthy bones and potassium helps control your heart rate and blood pressure by countering the effects of sodium (salt) in your diet.

Asparagus anyone?

Did you know that a simple red pepper is stuffed full of vitamin C? Did you know that vitamin C boosts your immune system?

And like Popeye have you had any spinach lately? Did you know that spinach is high in iron? And that iron is required by your body to make red blood cells and to help you breathe in sufficient oxygen? Spinach is also a rich source of omega-3 fatty acids and thus can help to lower your blood pressure and help with depression.[ix] It is not even that expensive. Make your mind up: a bottle of sugary fizz or a bag of spinach?

Spinach is Popeye's friend; make it yours too.

Make friends with all vegetables. Get to know them and what they do on your health's behalf.

Make friends with cabbage, cauliflower, courgette and cucumber.

Make friends with beetroot, beans and broccoli.

Make friends with potatoes, peas and parsnips.

Pack them on your plate every evening from now to infinity and beyond.
Be like me: become a born again vegetable eater.

Proclaim it to the world.

Say after me: vegetables are my friends.

Now dust down your boots. We're about to go walking...

These boots are made for walking

One of the first records I ever bought was Nancy Sinatra's These Boots Are Made for Walking.

One summer holiday from school the local kids and I organised an informal charity fundraising event to save our local church from closure. We asked the neighbours if there was anything they could contribute for us to sell. The neighbours, of course, were only too willing to part with unwanted household goods. Either that or we were just very charming children!

Their generosity for the cause of the church was incredible: cutlery, china, beautiful glasses, towels, coasters, lamp shades, various other assorted bric-a-brac and vinyl records. This was way before CDs and DVDs. Vinyl was cool man, seriously cool.

I had my eye on These Boots Are Made for Walking by Nancy Sinatra and made an early personal purchase. I couldn't wait to get home to play it and when I did it was at full volume.

I can still hear it in my mind all these years later:

> "You keep saying you've got something for me, something you call love but confess..."

I'm in heaven just imaging it as I write.

Nancy Sinatra: what a voice, perfect word emphasis and intonation too. And her boots – wow!

And as kids all summer we used to run about from early morning to late night with obligatory pit stops for lunch and dinner and only then because our parents yelled at us if we didn't.

They were halcyon days for sure.

The sun never stopped shining and we never stopped running about, playing tennis when Wimbledon was on, football when the World Cup was on, and cricket to keep one of the boys who visited from London happy. Then there were games of British Bulldogs where you had to cross the street from one pavement to the other without being caught. We sprinted, twisted and turned; every body movement and every range of speed and flexibility was on show.

We were kids, doing what kids do best: running, playing, eating a little and sleeping deeply until we could get up and do it all over again the next day.

For some reason as I grew up and became an adult all of that exercise became a thing of the past. I had to force myself to go out running and walking. I'm sure that happens to many adults. We have other demands placed upon us and exercise is not one of them so we drop it or just forget about it and as a life pattern it becomes a thing of the past, something we just no longer do.

Is that you?

I bet it is.

It just happens doesn't it?

You get a car or an office job in the city and kapow: little to no exercise other than walking to the car or to the vending machine for a coffee or the shops for lunch.

Somehow as adults it just happens. We slow down. Get less active. And it is the worst thing ever. Our all-round health depends on exercise.

Do you recall what Sir Harry Burns, Scotland's chief medical officer, said in my introduction? Just in case you have forgotten, he said that a lack of exercise is as damaging to our health as smoking, alcohol abuse and diabetes combined.

Staggering is it not?

It blew me away the first, second, third and fourth time I read it too.

Dr David Agus, author of A Short Guide to a Long Life, and a cancer expert to boot, notes that as far back at the 4th century BC Hippocrates said that "Walking is a man's best friend."[x]

Let me tell you: if it was good enough for Hippocrates it is good enough for you and me.

Indeed, if you have high blood pressure it is one of the few exercises you can do that won't overly stress your heart; instead, it will help get you slowly fit and aid blood pressure reduction in the process.

Now that sounds like a win-win doesn't it?

So that was why I dusted down my old waking boots and decided to hit the daily trail.

It is one of the best decisions I have ever made.

I love the fresh air in my lungs. My nose clears, my ears pop and my heart begins to beat anew. Warmth comes to my hands and toes; a small sweat dampens my shirt. My face begins to glow and it is as if I take in the energy from the trees and grassland that I walk across, becoming one with nature, shedding the stress and the worries, becoming the fit, healthy man I know I can once again be.

I know that sounds vaguely poetical but it is how I feel when I walk.

When I started my walking I did it at pace but as I collated my pulse reading with each blood pressure measurement I was becoming discouraged as my pulse was rising and falling. Indeed, it was going up and down like a fiddler's elbow.

What the heck was going on?

It didn't seem to make sense.

It was at this juncture my sister suggested I get a heart rate monitor to walk "in-zone."

I was sceptical.

I mean seriously it is only walking. Why the heck would I need a piece of technology to help me out?

Anyway, she is my big sister so I did as advised and bought a Beurer PM62 heart rate monitor. The Beurer PM62 was my choice and I have to say I am more than happy with its German engineering: it is solid, reliable and very functional.

Thank God for sisters eh?

She then kindly sent me a copy of Matt Robert's Fitness for Life Manual. It is an awesome book, full of eating and exercise advice. The best one for me was about heart rate training zones.

I'm going to explain this in the next chapter but for now dust down your old hiking boots and schedule time aside for a daily walk.

In my case I am lucky that I work from home. I schedule my walk to coincide with my son coming home from school. I meet him at the local railway station and we walk the last stretch home together with chocolate wrappers still stuffed inside his blazer pocket.

So, make time for walking my friend.

Do whatever it takes to ensure a daily routine.

If like my home town of Glasgow it rains a lot where you live make sure you have waterproof jackets and trousers. As the great comedian Billy Connolly once said: "In Scotland, there is no such thing as bad weather - only the wrong clothes."

Get out there. Get active. Recall your childhood and the energy you used to expend each and every day until you became a sedentary adult office worker or car driver.

Go on, do it.

Just tie up the laces of your boots and set off.

It is easy: one step, another step, and another...

The doctors say 30 minutes of walking at least five times a week should be your aim. Me? I walk for an hour+ each day because I love walking. That is 7+ hours of exercise every week. To be precise: 7+ hours more than I did before FAT BOB SLIM changed my life.

...and another step, and another step...

Why not listen to some music on your travels?

...and another step, and another step...

Where is Nancy Sinatra when you need her?

One, two, three all-together now:

"These boots were made for walking, and that's just what they'll do..."

You have to walk "in-the-zone" FAT BOB!

When I started walking at first I went at it hell-for-leather. It was my typical walking pace: full speed ahead. Perhaps it was a hang-over from days gone by when I was a regular runner and had lung bursting energy. More likely, it was the outcome of my frenetic working lifestyle, and a thing I learned from years of hard labour in the corporate arena: you've got to be fast or be nowhere.

Some just call it being stressed out.

The stressed out camp turned out to be spot-on.

If you are stressed my friend I hope you are taking note?

I'll tell you how to take your blood pressure and heart rate (pulse) readings in the next chapter. In the meantime, let me tell you that an adult should have a resting pulse of between 60 and 100 beats per minute. The lower your reading the fitter you are.

My resting pulse readings were shooting up and down like a fiddler's elbow. They ranged from 70 to 100 and sometimes more. Indeed, the faster I walked, in my frenzied way, the worse my resting pulse became. Up and down, up and down: it was all over the place and at the high end too, and worse than that it was on a rising trajectory.

I knew that was pretty bad.

I had expected that the more I exercised the stronger my heart would become. Improved fitness would surely follow all of this daily fast-paced walking over fields, along paths and up hills. But it didn't.

What the heck was going on?

If I am being honest it worried me.

It was obvious I was stressing myself even more than I needed but I hadn't a clue whether this would sort itself out naturally over the weeks ahead with improved fitness and weight loss or not.

Then my sister revealed that she walked with a heart rate monitor to help her gauge and improve her fitness levels. She has always been health conscious and suggested that I get one too. She even sent me a copy of Matt Robert's Fitness for Life Manual.[xi] That sort of kindness motivated me to find out what the heck was going on.

And, I needed to know.

Stressing your heart just isn't good.

I explored my options and purchased a Beurer PM62 heart rate monitor. The monitor consists of a chest strap that measures my heart rate as I walk and a watch that picks up the signal the chest strap transmits so I can see what is happening minute by minute as I look at my wrist.

The watch is a great device. It relays my heart rate as I walk and allows me to set a low and high zone in which to work out, otherwise known as working "in-the-zone."

More of this in a second...

The fitness and medical guys, not to mention my sister, were way ahead of me with "in-the-zone" training. I'd never even heard of it. I once heard David Blaine, the illusionist and endurance artist, talk about how he got "in-the-zone" so he could hold his breath for a prolonged spell under water. I got the idea. Being calm, reducing his heart rate, not allowing extraneous thoughts to enter his mind, to be quiet, still, focused.

So, I read up about "in-the-zone" training.

In essence it is simple and the difference it has made to my resting heart rate is impressive.

In order to work effectively and burn fat your heart rate, when you exercise, has to be between 65% and 85% of your maximum heart rate (MHR).[xii] Your MHR is given by this formula: 220 less your age. So, if like me you have reached the ripe old age of 50 it is 220 − 50 = 170. Thus 65% of my MHR is 110.5

and 85% is 144.5. As long as I work in-between these two figures I am strengthening my heart and most importantly I am not stressing it through manic exercise.

You have to walk "in-the-zone" FAT BOB!

After programming my heart rate monitor watch with my low and high measurements so it could keep me "in-the-zone" I found walking to be a really strange experience. Instead of rushing as I walked I was being told by my heart rate monitor to slow down. It was as if it was relaxing me, reminding me that I was overdoing it, stressing my heart, it was time to exercise but to take it easy as I did so.

And sure enough as I got better at working "in-the-zone" my resting heart rate began to level off. The horrible ups and downs became a thing of the past; the upward trajectory began to flatten and less than three weeks later it demonstrated a slight downward movement. As I write this I have reduced my resting pulse from its peak by a staggering 26% and the trend remains downwards.

One of the things I noticed, and I'm sure you will too, is that as you get fitter you have to work harder on your walks to stay "in-the-zone." At first, I was "in-the-zone" just walking up the hill outside my house on the way to the park. By the top of the hill I was easily out of the zone. The first few walks I was out of the zone about one third of the time – not great. But as I got fitter, walk after walk after walk, it was obvious my heart was becoming stronger and with effort rarely did I exceed my high limit of 85% of MHR.

Feeling more confident of myself and with my blood pressure steadily falling I decided to follow the advice in Matt Robert's Fitness for Life Manual: in particular, the advice in his walking programme to build endurance and stamina.

To build endurance Matt says I need to walk at a steady pace for an extended period of time. He suggests warming up for 4 minutes until I am at 75% of MHR (a pulse for me of 127.5) and then to maintain that pace for 20 minutes before cooling down by slowing my pace for 4 minutes until I am back to my resting rate.

To build stamina Matt says I need to walk for short periods at high intensity and alternate these with periods of low intensity. He suggests 4 minutes to warm up to 65% of MHR (a pulse for me of 110.5) and then walk at that pace for 2 minutes, then work up to 80% of MHR (a pulse for me of 136) and walk at that pace for 2 minutes. I then alternate between the two 5 times to give my heart a work-out.

As I write this I am in the process of trying out this endurance and stamina "in-the-zone" training. I will continue to measure and plot my resting pulse with each blood pressure reading to see what difference it makes i.e. will it lower my pulse, make me fitter, and encourage my heart to work less? If it does then it too should have a very positive effect on my blood pressure and weight loss. Thus far, 2 months in, I have moved from having a poor resting pulse to a higher than average resting pulse and now on to an average resting pulse and the trend is continuing downwards. I expect to have a better than average pulse within weeks. I am proud of that. I might not be in the "athlete" category[xiii] but I am getting fitter every day and my heart's fitness level is improving strongly in the right direction – a better than average resting pulse rate is now beckoning. I could never have dreamed of that when I first started out on FAT BOB SLIM.

So stick with it my friend.

Keep the faith.

And just remember this one thing:

You have to walk "in-the-zone" FAT BOB!

You also have to learn to eat three square meals a day as I am about to tell you...

Three square meals a day

When I was a child my mother served three square meals a day. That was how I learned to eat. We sat at the table as a family and her freshly prepared homemade food was served with steam rising from the plate. It is a memory I cherish to this day.

But something happened as I got older and it wasn't for the better: snacking became the norm.

Just a wee biscuit here, just a wee croissant there, and a "Why not try one of my buttered scones?" temptations everywhere!

But level with me: do you stop at one biscuit?

Do you put a nice bit of strawberry jam on your scone and maybe even some whipped cream too?

Or do you delude yourself by eating "healthy" oat and nut bars that have usually been dipped in honey and sugar with a smidgeon of chocolate coating too?

Maybe even just a wee cup of soup to warm you on a cold morning?

Or perhaps the call of the coffee shop for elevenses is too much and a latte beckons along with a wee treat i.e. some chocolate tiffin, to keep you rolling along?

I recall as a kid watching TV and seeing these cool American actors stopping off here and there, grabbing a quick burger, hotdog or doughnut as they went about their business, sipping take-away coffees like there was no tomorrow. For a wee boy across the Atlantic in downtown Glasgow where such things as take-away food hardly existed it was mesmerizingly cool, awesomely so. In fact it made me want to be able to do the same sort of thing. I'm pretty sure by the proliferation of take-away food in Glasgow today that I wasn't alone in my thought about how cool it looked.

But the big downside to all of this snacking is that we now eat whenever we want. Something to pep us up, something to keep us going, something to offer some comfort, a quick fix of sugar and fat to help us make it through yet another boring day at work.

Right?

We have lost the three square meals a day structure our parents introduced us to.

We have, quite simply, become 24/7 snackaholics!

If that is you then you might as well be honest and say out loud right now: "I am a 24/7 snackaholic!"

According to Dr Michael Mosley, compared to 30 years ago, we are eating around 180 calories per day more in snacks. We also now eat an extra 120 calories at regular mealtimes.[xiv]

Snacking it seems "just whets the appetite."[xv]

You might roll your eyes now and say "Well, so what?" I know I did when I used to hear this sort of stuff. But when calories, the measure of energy contained within our foods, were explained to me the penny at last dropped.

Snacking helps you put on weight and quickly too.

Let me explain:

All things being equal the average woman needs to eat around 1,940 calories per day; for men the figure is 2,550 calories. And, for every extra 3,500 calories you consume above your body's requirements you will gain a pound in weight.[xvi] In other words snacking and eating more calories with regular meals easily piles on additional pounds. For example: 180 calories each day in snacks alone will add an extra pound to your weight every 3 weeks.

Amazed? I was. But no more. And neither should you be.

It is simple: snacking piles on the pounds and is not required to maintain a healthy body.

So why snack?

On my FAT BOB SLIM regime I learned this lesson quickly and so adopted the three square meals each day philosophy to eating immediately. As it turned out it was a great first step towards understanding and effectively managing fasting - a calorie restricted day, something I will turn to in the next chapter.

If you can learn to eat three square meals a day without resorting to snacking you are demonstrating the ideal level of self-control required to lose weight. The best thing is that when it comes to regular meal times you will feel that you enjoy and value your food more than you have done in many a long year.

That was certainly the case for me.

I recall going the whole first morning of my three square meals a day week drinking only hot water and tea with a slice of lemon. My breakfast porridge with raspberries was delicious and filling but a wee biscuit, maybe a packet of crisps at 11am were serious temptations.

I made it through to lunchtime and had an amazing wholemeal bread and salmon sandwich with tomatoes and beetroot on the side. The taste of such simple food was hard to describe. Let me just say it was a sensation my taste buds had long forgotten. It was a bit like sitting down at the table as a child with my mother again and savouring every mouthful of her homemade cooking. I ate my sandwich slowly, tasting every mouthful and texture, mixing in a cherry tomato and a slice of beetroot to add to the joy I was experiencing. I followed that sandwich with an orange and a banana. For some reason they too tasted like proper fruit. In truth, that afternoon the temptation to snack had gone. It was as if my brain knew to look forward to its evening meal of lean frying steak with red peppers and onions on a bed of Savoy cabbage. Even typing that just now has made me salivate but I am not tempted to snack because I know that snacking ruins the taste of the lovely food I have planned for my evening meal. And if it can work for a FAT BOB I am certain it can work for you too. You just need to be prepared to give it a go and let the magic begin...

So my message to you is very simple: quit snacking and commit to three square meals a day from now on.

Give it a go.

Get through your first week without snacking and you will never look back; food will become not an obsession but something to savour at regular mealtimes.

Better still, when you walk past that vending machine in the office you won't hear its seductive voice: "Hi there FAT BOB, haven't seen you in some time..." You won't be tempted either. In fact, if you are anything like me, you will feel pity for the poor folks who have been seduced by the snack industry, the ones piling on the pounds and dangerously raising their blood pressure in the process. You will look on with new eyes, you will yield not to temptation; instead, you will metaphorically rise to majestic heights knowing your health is all the better for your courage to desist.

Courage 1: Snack Industry 0.

Begin today.

Make a commitment to eating three square meals a day from here to infinity and beyond...

Know that your regular meals will taste so much better when you stick to this approach to eating.

And, once you have managed this three square meals a day approach to eating you are ready to begin your first day of fasting.

More about this in the next chapter.

Fasting: lose weight the easy way

I want to start this chapter with a confession.

It is the sort of admission that defies logic.

But it happens to be true.

And it is part of the reason why my FAT BOB SLIM regime is SO successful.

Do you want to know what it is?

Go on, take a guess.

No?

Okay, let me just blurt it out: I DON'T COUNT CALORIES.

There, I've said it and immediately feel all the better for it.

The thought of weighing food every day from here until when I meet my maker drives me nuts.

I mean seriously, do you think our cave dwelling, hunter gathering ancestors whipped out a set of Salter scales just before tucking into a leg of roast boar?

No, I didn't think so!

Yet these same ancestors we know weren't fat. Obesity wasn't a problem for them but finding food was. Their bodies and ours too have been wired for feast and fast.[xvii]

Yet in our modern Western economies food is, for most, in glorious abundance. And the net result is that we feast, feast, feast. We don't call it that. We refer to it innocently as overeating, junk food and snacking. But in essence it is the same thing: taking in more energy than our bodies require.

In other words a feast!

And, of course, the more you feast the fatter you become.

Have you spotted the one thing missing from all of this?

Yes, you've got it: we never fast!

Yet, fasting is increasingly being shown to be good for the body. It is said to lower blood sugar (and thus the risk of developing diabetes) and assist the body's natural repair genes.

I'm not qualified to say whether it does or it doesn't.

But I can say this for certain: fasting has helped me to shed in excess of 40 lbs over a 4 month window without once having had to worry about counting calories.

I skip lunch 2 days each week and the weight drops off.

Honestly, it is as simple as that.

It is so good I will say it again for emphasis:

I skip lunch 2 days each week and the weight drops off.

Do I get hungry?

Do I get lightheaded?

Do I get headaches?

Do my energy levels dip?

Am I tempted to snack?

In truth, I can get slightly hungry, particularly as I get closer to dinner time. I make sure I drink lots throughout the day so I don't get headaches. And as long as I keep busy and not fixated on food my energy levels are fine and snacking seems unimportant.

It really is that simple.

Let me be clear, just in case you are worried: my skipping lunch is not a heavy duty fast.

I eat breakfast before work and don't eat again until about 7:30pm. In other words I fast over an eleven hour period on two days of the week. And during my fast I drink fluid, lots of water and herbal teas but never alcohol.

And the great thing is: this type of fasting is not that challenging if you have first become accustomed to eating 3 square meals a day.

You simply have to try it to believe me.

Further, I actually enjoy my fast days. Firstly, I feel lighter, fresher, and more alert on a fast day. And, secondly, my food in the evening is simply THE BEST. It is mouth-wateringly delicious. My taste buds come to life. The sensation has to be experienced to be believed...

Fasting is everywhere, and it has ancient, religious roots too.

In exploring the subject I have discovered there are many varieties of fasting: the Full Fast is where you drink fluids only over a number of specified days – best supervised; the Daniel Fast, a religious one, where no meat, sweet or bread is eaten, though fluids, fruits and vegetables are allowed along with prayer, reflection and worship; the 3 Day Fast – this can be a Full Fast, a Daniel Fast or where one item of food is given up; and the Partial Fast from 6:00am to 3:00pm which can be a Full Fast, a Daniel Fast or where you give up one item of food.[xviii]

Permutation upon permutation...

It all seems endless doesn't it?

Sometimes you will hear it referred to as a detox rather than a fast.

It goes on and on...

But the essence is always the same:

On a FAST day you consume far fewer calories and drink far more fluid than on a normal day.

Simple isn't it?

So are you up for the challenge?

Are you regularly eating three square meals a day without snacking?

Do you want to see the weight drop off?

If so then your first fast day is beckoning you to step forward.

It is inviting you to follow a new lifestyle.

One that will see the pounds drop off.

One that will make you feel fresh, light and mentally alert.

One that will transform your health.

One that will reduce your risk of developing diabetes.

One that will lower your blood pressure.

Fasting will become a new way of life. It will feel like the right thing to do. It will refresh and revitalise you. Your energy will soar despite the lack of calorie intake. It is one of the great paradoxes you simply have to experience to believe.

Fasting is now my counterbalance.

If I eat too much, it corrects that imbalance for me.

If I feel full it makes me light again.

If my spirits are down, it lifts them.

And all the time it is acting as my counterbalance it is also enabling me to lose weight and slash my blood pressure. It is such a fabulous thing to do. I wholeheartedly recommend it despite my intense cynicism at the outset. I learned to open up and have been amazed at the outcome.

My wife, who is equally cynical, now joins me on one of my weekly fast days. Recently she announced that instead of fasting one day each week she would increase it to two days. And her experience of this: "The weight comes off much more quickly and my stomach feels less bloated." These are her words, not mine.

Does she feel hungry on a fast day?

Yes, but not so much that she has to break into a snack.

We fast together.

We are a team.

We support one another.

We go walking.

We get involved so that our missed lunch is forgotten.

We drink herbal teas.

We shop. I write books and she edits. We do good deeds.

We plan our evening meal in advance.

We know it is something to look forward to: salmon and roast vegetables.

The time passes almost unnoticed.

Dinner time arrives and our food is delicious. We relish it like no other. We had taken food for granted; we had become immune to its taste, but no longer.

My friend, the next step is waiting for you too.

Fasting is inviting you to come forward with open arms. If you have dumped the junk food, if you are eating three square meals a day without snacking, you are ready to accept its offer.

Embrace your fast day.

Be prepared for it.

Plan what you will eat for breakfast and dinner in advance.

Know what you will drink during the day and make sure you take sufficient to prevent dehydration and headaches.

Keep busy.

Do your walk at lunchtime. Let the time pass and keep focused. If hunger tries to trick you sip water to keep it at bay. If you feel an irresistible urge to snack remember how much it will ruin your appetite. And why would you want to do that when the taste of heavenly food will be yours in the evening?

Yield not to temptation...

You can do it.

You can do it and make fasting an intrinsic part of your FAT BOB SLIM lifestyle.

Commit to it.

Commit to it two days each week.

Commit to it and you will see the weight drop off.

FAT BOB is a SLIM BOB because of fasting.

Give it a go my friend.

Stick with it.

Make it a way of life.

As the weeks pass the weight will drop off.

And like me you'll no longer be a FAT BOB; you'll be a SLIM BOB instead. Now that has to be worth a shot, right?

Get rid of the SALT!

How much salt do you eat in a day?

Any idea?

Take a guess. Go on...

According to Blood Pressure UK "80% of the salt you eat every day is 'hidden' in the...foods you eat."[xix]

Is that not astonishing?

It also helps explain why so many adults have developed high blood pressure. FAT BOB SLIM included. Yes, me. It is just so darned easy to sleep walk into bad health.

But more of this in a minute...

The NHS (National Health Service in the UK) advises that adults should consume no more than 6g of salt each day – that is about one full teaspoon.[xx] You will often see salt and sodium mentioned on the packaging that comes with food. Even with a science degree it confused the life out of me: salt and sodium, are they not one in the same? It is easy to imagine they are but they are not.

For simplicity, the relationship is as follows:

Salt = Sodium × 2.5

Thus 6g of salt = 2.4g of sodium.

Capiche?

Salt in my porridge, salt on my chips, salt rubbed into beef sandwiches...it soon adds up. And dangerously so I'm afraid. The net result is high blood pressure and serious health implications you most certainly don't want. Unless, of course, you have a perverted sense of humour and find the thought of having a stroke or heart disease to be jaw-breakingly funny pastimes?

No, I didn't think so...

And the frightening thing is that most of the salt is hidden in the foods we commonly consume without giving them a second thought. Foods like bacon, cheese, smoked meat, smoked fish, anything smoked in fact, pizza, tinned and packaged soup, ready meals out the freezer cabinet at the supermarket, fast foods from the proliferation of fast food joints in the high street, crisps in the vending machines at work, soy sauce at the Chinese restaurant, stock cubes we so innocently make our healthy vegetable soups with, bread that we dip in to our "healthy" soup, breakfast cereals (yes seriously; they might be high in vitamins and promoted as being good for kids but sadly they are also dangerously high in salt), mayonnaise, anchovies, sardines and the tasty, lip-smacking olives I am tempted to over indulge in at my local restaurant to name but a limited few of the salty food culprits.

That is even before I reach for the salt cellar...

It is noted that most people in the UK consume 8.1g of salt each day – that is 3.24g of sodium.[xxi] The Institute of Medicine in America advises everyone to limit daily sodium intake to just 2.3g.[xxii] That is 0.1g lower than recommended in the UK. Further, they stress that adequate sodium intake is just 1.5g per day and that that is what you and I should be aiming to consume if we want to reduce our blood pressure and the horrible health risks like stroke and heart disease associated with it.

So let me just repeat that:

Adults should aim for 1.5g of sodium per day: equivalent to 3.75g of salt per day.

When I had my blood pressure checked by the nurse she advised me to reduce my salt intake. She didn't say by how much; just that I should reduce it. So that is why I mention the figures above. You may experience the same at your health centre and leave none the wiser where salt and sodium are concerned.

On my FAT BOB SLIM regime I have tried hard to reduce and keep to a minimum my daily salt and sodium intake.

I have been astonished at the number of things I used to eat that are high in salt. I can still eat them, of course, but as I never exceed my 1.5g of sodium per day it just means I will deprive myself of other tasty things and I think that is verging on stupidity given the range of alternative options available to me. So instead, I have learned which foods are lower in salt and I eat them in preference and then bulk my plate out with healthy vegetables.

It is pretty simple and it works.

So I eat lean meat like chicken and also buy frying steaks which are mostly protein, with some fats but incredibly are super low in salt. I also eat lots more fish than I have ever done before. A word of warning, watch out for smoked fish, and some tinned sardines and anchovies as they are very, very salty.

Just saying...

The best advice is simply to read the labels on the food before you buy them. They usually tell you how much salt or sodium equivalent there is per 100g of serving. Figure out how much salt or sodium will be in your serving and plan your 3 square meals a day accordingly so that the total does not exceed 1.5g of sodium or 3.75g of salt. Once you have done this a few times you won't need to bother with the calculations. You will be on automatic healthy pilot mode and your blood pressure will thank you for your kindness. Your overworked kidneys will be more than grateful too.

FAT BOB SLIM measures his blood pressure twice each day: 3 times in the morning and 3 times in the evening, each reading is 3 minutes apart. I sit in silence for 5 minutes to relax before the first reading, and the overall measurements are averaged. Early on I noticed that my blood pressure spiked each time I ate salty food like bacon or tinned soup or took a slice of "healthy topping" pizza. It was only then I was able to appreciate the effect of salty food on my blood pressure. My visit to the nurse came a stage later. That's life as they say.

But unlike me you don't have to try to figure this out for yourself instead, just stick within the recommended limit of 1.5g sodium or 3.75g salt each day and, if your blood pressure is anything like mine, it will start to reduce and respond more than favourably in the weeks ahead.

Knowing the damage that salt can do I am always on the look-out for statistics that highlight this and help make the dangers of over consumption more obvious.

Here is one statement that does it for me:

It is said that if the average American reduced their sodium intake by 1.2g per day "...it would prevent about 90,000 new cases of Coronary Heart Disease, about 49,000 strokes, 76,000 heart attacks, and 68,000 deaths from all causes each year."[xxiii]

If you are one of my American readers make sure you are not included in the above statistics. The same statistics will apply in the UK too I am sure and in Scotland in particular with our obesity epidemic not far behind the land of the free, the dear old USA.

So my friend PLEASE just do as I say in the title of this chapter and Get rid of the SALT!

It is so easy to sleepwalk into bad health.

It is so easy to consume too much salt.

It is so easy to develop high blood pressure.

It is then only a matter of time before heart disease, heart attack, stroke and death are upon you.

So PLEASE dear friend, I beg you: Get rid of the SALT!

Eat well, live longer...

The NHS has a change4life website that says if you eat well and move more you should live longer.[xxiv]

"Eat well, Move more, Live longer"

My friend, that is FAT BOB SLIM in a nutshell.

If you consume lots of fat, excess sugar and salt expect to gain weight and sleepwalk into serious illness.

I should know – I did!

But put on your walking boots and eat healthily and the tide begins to turn. The healthy you reemerges from the shadows.

I know about that too – it does!

But before I go further with this healthy eating lark I have a confession to make:

"FAT BOB SLIM can't cook!"

In truth I am a very ordinary chef.

I am an embarrassment to my late mother's memory. I cannot even pretend to imitate her depth and breadth of culinary expertise. She was phenomenal: the fish cakes on Thursday after school sports, the steam rising from vegetable soup served on a cold winter's evening, and glazed lemon meringue pie straight from the oven on a Sunday afternoon...

What was not to love and admire about her cooking?

Me?

I am of a generation where no one taught me to cook, make or prepare meals. They didn't teach me and neither was it expected that I would want or need to learn.

That is what mothers and wives did!

My cooking skills, limited as they are, I learned through books and TV series like Delia Smith's and Rick Stein's.

But as a time-limited worker and father I found that buying pizza was easier. There must be many people out there like that.

Goodness knows how many men and women I meet these days who confess:

"I'm rotten at cooking – I either eat out or buy a take-away."

My friend that statement is merely an excuse for not making the effort to cook and eat healthily.

I know.

To my cost, I know.

It was my excuse too.

Mother, I am sorry that I didn't learn more from you. I should have taken the opportunity when you were in your cooking prime, I should have learned how to cook healthily.

Instead, as I got older and lived by myself, I found it was easy to tuck into take-away pizza and slurp a cool can of foaming lager straight from the fridge.

It became a habit.

But there comes a time when you need to demonstrate self-respect.

Do you want to sleepwalk into illness and obesity or are you going to make a fist of healthy eating?

I tell you this: healthy eating is simple. So bloody simple I wonder how I managed to avoid doing it for so long.

FAT BOB SLIM has had to take a long, hard look at himself in the mirror.

Cave men and women weren't lazy.

Cave men and women were slim as a result.

Cave women collected fruits and vegetables.

Cave men collected protein: meats and fish.

Together cave men and women ate healthily.

Cave children followed suit.

Like a cave child FAT BOB SLIM has learned to do that too.

And, better late than never!

I'd never make a contestant on MasterChef, and I can't come close to the great food my mother used to prepare but each day my plates are now packed with vegetables and healthy food, and the difference it has made to my body is incredible.

So at the sake of repeating myself:

> "If a 220 lbs pizza munching, lager swilling Glaswegian can do it – so can you!"

My friend, get your apron on and let's get cooking.

Below are my collection of breakfast, lunch and dinner recipes. They are simple, tasty and healthy.

They will help you to shed the pounds and slash your blood pressure – that's my kind of eating, make it yours too.

Enjoy!

Breakfast

Scots Porridge & fruit topping

Ingredients:

½ a cup of porridge
A handful of raspberries
A handful of blackberries
A cup of skimmed milk

Method:

Put porridge in bowl
Add the cup of skimmed milk and stir
Place bowl in microwave on high for 90 seconds
Remove bowl and add some milk and stir to maintain moisture
Return bowl to microwave for 60 seconds
Remove
Top with raspberries and blackberries
Pour some milk on top

Serve with a cup of tea, herbal tea or coffee

Notes:

Ideal for fast days
No salt added
Vary toping with fruit in season
Strawberries in summer are awesome
On non-fast days serve with a piece of fruit e.g. an orange

Poached eggs on toast

Ingredients:

2 medium sized eggs
1 medium slice of wholemeal bread
A stalk of vine tomatoes (5 or 6 tomatoes)
A small stick of celery

Method:

Toast bread
Poach eggs
Serve eggs on toast
Serve tomatoes and celery on the side
Sprinkle pepper over eggs

Serve with a cup of tea, herbal tea or coffee

Notes:

Ideal for fast day
No butter or spread used on toast
Eggs can be scrambled or fried in a small amount of olive oil to add variety
On non-fast days add a piece of fruit e.g. an orange

Muesli, yoghurt and fruit mélange

Ingredients:

45g of muesli
Natural yoghurt
A small handful of strawberries
A small handful of blueberries
A small handful of blackberries

Method:

Add muesli to bowl
Add yoghurt to muesli as required
Top with a mixture of strawberries, blueberries and blackberries

Serve with a cup of tea, herbal tea or coffee

Notes:

In summer drizzle on a little runny honey for a treat

Mushroom & tomato frittata

Ingredients:

2 medium eggs
A handful of cherry tomatoes
A large handful of chestnut mushrooms
1 small onion
A handful of spinach

Method:

Preheat grill
Add a drizzle of olive oil to omelette pan and heat on hob
Break eggs in to a bowl and beat
Dice tomatoes, mushroom and onion and add to heated omelette pan
Season with mixed herbs
Add some black pepper
Allow to cook and briefly stir as you go
Add the beaten eggs and spinach to the omelette pan and allow all contents to cook
Place omelette pan under grill and allow to rise and finish off cooking
Serve on plate

Serve with a cup of tea, herbal tea or coffee

Notes:

Ideal for a fast day.

On non-fast days grate strong cheddar cheese over omelette pan after adding spinach
Can also be served as a lunch on non-fast days

Lunch

FAT BOB's amazing no mayo tuna sandwich

Ingredients:

½ tin of tuna in springwater
2 slices of medium wholemeal bread
Spread (low salt)
½ red onion
A sprig of parsley
5 vine tomatoes
5 pitted black olives
½ a lemon
A handful of spinach
2 small beetroots

Method:

Dice red onion and tomatoes
Finely chop parsley
Place above in a bowl with the tuna and mix
Squeeze in some lemon juice
Season with black pepper
Apply spread to bread
Serve tuna mix on bread and make sandwich
Serve with a side of spinach leaves, chopped beetroot and olives

Serve with a cup of tea, herbal tea, coffee or a tall glass of water with a drop of lime cordial

Notes:

An ideal non-fast day lunch

Simple cheese & tomato omelette

Ingredients:

1 small onion
2 medium sized tomatoes
2 medium sized eggs
Strong cheddar cheese

Method:

Break eggs into a bowl and beat
Quarter the tomatoes
Dice the onion
Drizzle a few drops of olive oil in an omelette pan
When warm add the onion and tomatoes and cook
Pour in the egg mix
Grate fine covering of cheese over the mix
Add some mixed herbs
Season with black pepper

Serve with a cup of tea, herbal tea, coffee or a tall glass of water with a drop of lime cordial

Follow with a banana and orange

Notes:

An ideal non-fast day lunch

Fried eggs on toast

Ingredients:

2 medium sized eggs
2 slices of wholemeal bread
A stalk of vine tomatoes
A handful of spinach leaves
2 small beetroots
5 black pitted olives
HP sauce

Method:

Heat frying pan with small glug of olive oil
Break eggs into pan and cook
Toast bread then apply spread
Serve eggs – one on each slice of toast
Add small covering of sauce to each egg
Serve with side salad of spinach, sliced beetroot, vine tomatoes and olives

Serve with a cup of tea, herbal tea, coffee or a tall glass of water with a drop of lime cordial

Follow with an apple and bunch of grapes

Notes:

An ideal non-fast day lunch

Vegetarian club sandwich

Ingredients:

3 slices of medium wholemeal bread
2 medium sized tomatoes
A handful of rocket leaves
1 small carrot
½ lemon
Olive oil
Reduced fat houmous

Method:

Toast bread
Medium slice the tomatoes
Peel and grate carrot
In a bowl mix the rocket and carrot and add a glug or two of olive oil and a squeeze of lemon juice
Spread houmous on one side of toast × 2 - spread houmous on both sides of middle slice of toast
On bottom layer of toast add ½ of the mix and top with tomato, then add the middle toast layer
On the middle toast layer add remainder of mix and top with tomato and final layer of toast, then cut diagonally and serve

Serve with a cup of tea, herbal tea or coffee and an orange

Notes:

An ideal non-fast day lunch

Dinner (Serves 3)

Mediterranean roast veg & salmon

Ingredients:

1 red pepper
1 yellow pepper
1 courgette (zucchini)
1 red onion
10 black pitted olives
15 vine tomatoes
Olive oil
3 salmon fillets

Method:

Slice courgette, peppers and onion
Add to baking tray
Add olives and tomatoes
Pour over a few glugs of olive oil
Sprinkle over some mixed herbs
Season with black pepper
Put in oven at gas mark 8 for 20 minutes
At 20 mins place salmon fillets in baking tray
Bake for a further 10 minutes and serve

Notes:

Ideal for a fast day
Great with haddock or cod too
On a non-fast day serve with baked potatoes – add a
slice of low salt butter

Follow with a pink grapefruit

Lean frying steak with red peppers & red onion on a bed of cabbage

Ingredients:

½ Savoy cabbage
1 large red pepper
1 large red onion
3 lean frying steaks

Method:

Slice the cabbage and steam in pan with lid for 10 minutes
Slice the red pepper
Dice the onion
Add to a frying pan with a glug of olive oil
Fry the pepper and onion briefly then add the steaks
Sprinkle some mixed herbs
Season with black pepper
Turn the steaks often until done
Add some water to prevent sticking
Drain the cabbage and serve on plate
Serve the steaks on the cabbage
Spoon over the red pepper and onion

Notes:

Ideal for a fast day
On a non-fast day serve with baked potatoes – add a slice of low salt butter
Make sure the steaks are low salt content
Follow with a pink grapefruit

Roast chicken & steamed veg

Ingredients:

1 oven ready chicken
1 onion
1 broccoli stalk
2 carrots

Method:

Place chicken on a roll of silver foil and add to a roasting pan
Chop onion and sprinkle over the chicken
Season with black pepper
Sprinkle over some mixed herbs
Drizzle over some olive oil
Wrap in the foil and add to an oven
Cook at temperature and time recommended for weight of chicken
After 1hr open the foil and spoon over the oil regularly until ready to serve
Prepare broccoli and carrots and add to a pan of boiling water and place on lid to steam
When chicken and vegetables are ready serve and enjoy

Notes:

Ideal for a fast day
On a non-fast day serve with baked potatoes
Read packaging on chicken to confirm salt content

Cod & broccoli surprise

Ingredients:

3 cod fillets
1 red pepper
1 red onion
A small slice of root ginger
1 stalk of broccoli

Method:

Steam the broccoli
Chop the pepper, onion and ginger then add to frying pan with a few drops of olive oil and toasted sesame oil
Add the cod fillets and sprinkle over some mixed herbs and season with black pepper
Turn the cod until ready
Serve on a plate with the broccoli and spoon over the red pepper and onion mix

Notes:

Ideal for a fast day
On a non-fast day serve with baked potatoes or small portion of rice
Instead of cod try salmon or haddock
Follow with a pink grapefruit

Food: what to be aware of?

Look out for the salt content and remain within limit.

On a fast day eat a small amount of protein e.g. chicken or fish, and pack the remainder of your plate with vegetables.

Potatoes are no longer categorised as a vegetable; instead, they are a source of carbohydrate, namely starch.

On fast days reduce the amount of carbohydrate that you eat. It is said that this helps to reduce your body's blood sugar level and chance of developing diabetes – assuming you don't already have it.

Alcohol is best avoided on fast days and minimised in general. It is full of calories and carbohydrates. It might just look like an innocent drink but it doesn't half help to pile on the pounds.

Another high calorie culprit is mayonnaise and dressings in general. Check out the labels before you pour. Try alternatives like drizzling on lemon juice or balsamic vinegar – these options are far better on calories and salt levels.

Blood pressure: measure it, control it, reduce it...

Do you know what blood pressure is?

Have you heard of systolic and diastolic blood pressure?

Do you know your actual systolic and diastolic blood pressure readings?

Do you understand what these readings are telling you?

I certainly didn't. And that is despite having a degree in science!

Indeed, I probably went for several years blissfully unaware my blood pressure readings were dangerously high.

I put my health at serious risk in the process.

I could have died.

Ignorance, as they say, is no defence in the face of death.

So in this chapter I'm going to tell you about blood pressure, what it is, how you measure it, how to control it, and most importantly of all, if your blood pressure is high, how to reduce it.

And the truth is, as my Hershey-handed son so often says as he rolls his eyes in disbelief at my technical incompetence: "It's easy peasy lemon squeezy daaaad!"

So if a FAT BOB can learn about blood pressure, what it is, how to control it, and how to reduce it then so can you.

Let me begin with the equivalent of a school boy's biology lesson:

When your heart beats it pumps blood around your body. The blood picks up oxygen from the lungs and transports this along with energy e.g. sugar, to the various cells and organs of the body so that they can function properly.

When your blood moves along the arteries that lead from the heart it is under pressure. It is metaphorically "kicked" along the arteries to ensure that it travels right around your system. Thankfully, there are also a series of valves in place to make sure your blood can't flow backwards. Clever stuff eh?

This "kicking" of the blood places pressure on the walls of your arteries. It is this pressure that is measured by your doctor. The maximum pressure with each heartbeat is known as systolic and the minimum is known as diastolic.

Got it?

Thus your doctor will tell you two numbers with each blood pressure reading. The first number is the systolic and the second number is the diastolic. It is also commonly written as one number over another e.g. 120/80, and simply said as: "120 over 80."

The unit of pressure measurement is in millimetres of mercury. The chemistry students amongst you, my son included, will know this is shortened to mm Hg: Hg is the symbol for mercury. But that doesn't really matter. What does matter, however, are the systolic and diastolic measurements from your readings and whether they are considered to be high or not.

Now, you may ask, as I did, why these numbers are important.

Let me continue with my beginner's biology lesson:

If your blood pressure is high then so is the pressure on your artery walls. If this pressure is high for too long it causes your arteries to harden and narrow. The result of this physical change is increased blood pressure known as hypertension: commonly referred to as high blood pressure. As in: "Oh God! FAT BOB SLIM has got high blood pressure."

Hypertension is known as the "silent killer."

It is simple: just like me, you won't know that you have it. There are few if any symptoms. Hence: the "silent killer" description. As I've said before, high blood pressure leads to heart attacks and strokes, and may cause kidney damage and a host of other potential nasties such as erectile dysfunction and blindness.

FAT BOB SLIM was just waiting to become FAT BOB HEART ATTACK, FAT BOB STROKE, and potentially FAT BOB EARLY DEATH...

The thought of that motivated me to take action: make sure it motivates you too. Substitute your name above in place of BOB and feel the need to act with some degree of urgency.

So there you have it. Now you know what blood pressure is and why it is so important to measure it and control it.

My friend: don't die of ignorance.

Let's take the next step together as I explain how to take and measure your blood pressure like a pro.

I started by buying an automatic blood pressure monitor. My son loved the thought of me ordering an electronic gadget he could get his mucky paws on. At my doctor's practice I had noted they used Omron blood pressure monitors so I got online and ordered one for myself. It wasn't that pricey. Thanks to Amazon it arrived the next morning. My son was hyper-excited as I opened the packaging to reveal the contents. He figured it all out for his old dad in next to no time. Thanks son, love you. For advice on which ones to purchase, ones that are validated and also respected by the medical community, look at Blood Pressure UK's website at www.bloodpressureuk.org It is well worth the view. The website also has a video telling you how to take a blood pressure reading. It is well worth watching this because I am about to explain this next.

Once your blood pressure monitor arrives read the instruction manual that comes with it, sit at the kitchen table and you are ready to begin by taking your first reading.

Yup, it's that simple.

Sit comfortably and upright in a hard backed chair. Apply the armband to your upper arm (left or right). It should be about two fingers' width up from the bend in your elbow and you should be able to slip at least one finger under the armband itself: it should be snug but not overly tight as you take your reading.

It is critical that your arm is at heart height when you take your readings.

Now, note the time and sit quietly for a full five minutes with your feet flat on the floor. Blood pressure should be taken in a calm state. Try to get rid of distraction and distracting thoughts in particular and don't talk or move as you take your reading. Also, make sure beforehand that you have been to the toilet and are comfortable. And never take a reading until at least 30 minutes after exercise, eating, smoking or drinking alcohol.

And if you smoke, sorry but you really need to quit for the sake of your and everybody else's health. End of!

Now, note down the time you were seated. Add five minutes to that and that will be when you take your first reading. You should be calm by that point. Add another three minutes and that will be your second reading and add another three minutes and that will be your third and final reading. Blood pressure is dynamic, it is never still, it goes up and down throughout the day, minute by minute and second by second, so three readings will give you a good working average.

To take your first reading all you will need to do is press the button on your automatic blood pressure monitor and it will do the rest. It will inflate the armband, monitor your systolic and diastolic blood pressure and your resting heart rate known simply as your pulse. If your monitor is anything like mine it will make things easy for you by displaying your readings on the screen.

Make a note of these three figures: systolic, diastolic and pulse.

Wait three more minutes to allow your arteries to return to normal and take your second reading.

Again, note your systolic, diastolic and pulse measurements.

Finally, wait three more minutes and take your third and final reading. Again noting your systolic, diastolic and pulse measurements.

Simple eh?

Here is a FAT BOB SLIM example table:

I sat at 8:42am. I relaxed and breathed slowly for 5 minutes with my blood pressure monitor armband applied. I took my first reading at 8:47am. I took my second reading at 8:50am. I took my third and final reading at 8:53am.

Time	8:47am	8:50am	8:53am
Systolic	102	100	98
Diastolic	71	73	72
Pulse	65	66	64

So, now you know what blood pressure is, why understanding it is important, and how to measure it like a pro.

I am proud of you!

But what do your readings tell you?

This is the important bit, the moment of truth: high blood pressure or not?

The table below indicates that if your systolic blood pressure is between 90 and 120 it is ideal. And, if your diastolic blood pressure is between 60 and 80 it too is ideal. If, however, your blood pressure is above these upper limits you need to act to reduce it. Capiche?

Systolic	Diastolic	Blood Pressure
<90	<60	Low
>90 <120	>60 <80	Ideal
>120 <140	>80 <90	Pre-High
>140	>90	High

FAT BOB SLIM's first home reading was 165/95. The subsequent plus one reading was 175/100. That is super high. It was rising. I needed to act and quickly too.

The advice given by the highly respected World Health Organization (WHO) and the International Society of Hypertension (ISH) is that home readings consistently above 135/85 are considered to represent high blood pressure.[xxv]

I'll say that again:

Home readings consistently above 135/85 are considered to represent high blood pressure.

Even if your blood pressure is in the pre-high level for either systolic or diastolic you need to take action to prevent yourself sleepwalking into high blood pressure and ill health. It is simply too easily done.

98

So, do you have high blood pressure?

Or are you in the pre-high blood pressure range?

If you are reading FAT BOB SLIM it is quite likely that you will fall into one or other of these ranges: that is what being overweight does to you, it is bad for your health.

If you have high blood pressure talk to your doctor. Lift the phone up and make an appointment. Whatever you do don't delay. Tell him about your blood pressure readings. Tell him about your FAT BOB SLIM plan to lose weight, exercise and cut out salt. Work with him to make sure your health is top priority.

I'm talking to you heart to heart here - no pun intended:

I was serious about reducing my blood pressure and weight. I was serious because of the risk to my health that went with it. I was serious because the thought of not being about to see my son grow up, to laugh my head off at his surreptitious ways where chocolate bar wrappers are concerned, to see his eager face as I unwrap the latest piece of technology he can play with, was too much, far too much responsibility to bear: I had no option other than to act.

As I write these lines I do so with a tear in my eye and one persistent thought:

99

"What if I hadn't acted?"

My earnest hope is that you WILL act.

My earnest hope is that you too will put your health first and shed a tear at the thought of the loved ones you could leave behind, the ones that make your life so special, so full of joy and inspiration. Yes, do it for you; do it for them too - JUST DO IT!

If you are really committed to this FAT BOB SLIM regime, if you really want to slash your blood pressure then stay tuned as I share how you can do so.

Are you ready for this?

Well, believe it or not if you have acted upon my advice in previous chapters you have already started. Yup! You read me correctly: you have already started. Pat yourself on the back. Well done!

Let me explain:

Have you dumped the junk food?

Do you eat three square meals a day and NO snacks?

And do you fast two days each week?

If so you have begun to reduce your daily calorie intake and weight. Bravo!

Have you got rid of the salt?

If you have reduced your salt intake you have begun to ease the pressure on your artery walls. Bravo!

Have you started to eat lots more vegetables?

If you have you are improving your all round health and wellbeing. Bravo!

Have you begun daily walking?

If you have your heart will be responding positively. Believe it or not it is silently thanking you and getting stronger each and every day you pound the streets, straddle the puddles, and climb the hills. Bravo!

All of the above have a positive impact on your weight and blood pressure. But it is early days and if you have just started monitoring your weight and blood pressure you might not see any perceptible improvements: stick with it, for, if you are anything like me, improvements will come as sure as night follows day.

Plot your systolic, diastolic and pulse measurements each day on the graph card that came with your monitor. Plot them on an Excel spreadsheet too. It doesn't have to be fancy, just sufficient for you to observe the trend when you plot a line diagram. I also plotted a moving average of each of these three measurements by taking the current and last two readings so that a clearer trend could be observed. You could do the same. It will be interesting to see where you are one week, two weeks, three weeks, a month, two months, three months on from the day you first started FAT BOB SLIM. I was amazed by it and I still am...

The experts say that "losing weight has the biggest effect on those who are overweight and already have hypertension."[xxvi]

In the next chapter I will introduce you to yoga breathing exercises. These too can help to significantly reduce your blood pressure. But for now let me note some statistics for you.

My first set of home blood pressure readings were an average 165/95. That is well above the WHO's 135/85 upper limit for home readings. I was consistently on the high side of the line. Yet, 60 days into FAT BOB SLIM and my average had reduced to an astonishing 106/74. That is comfortably within the ideal blood pressure range for both systolic and diastolic. In fact it is a 36% reduction for systolic and a 22% reduction for diastolic. That is simply awesome and beyond my wildest expectations. In truth, I never thought I would get there at all let alone in 60 days. At the outset my readings were high and getting higher. I knew I had high blood pressure. The more I fretted over this the worse it got. But I stayed the course, knowing that the health experts were right, knowing that I needed to lose weight, modify my diet, do exercise and control my stress.

I also knew that my FAT BOB SLIM regime was the answer.

Now, let me repeat what the experts say in case you missed it:

"Losing weight has the biggest effect on those who are overweight and already have hypertension."

In my opinion everything else, the walking, the dumping of the junk food, the 3 square meals a day, the fasting, the reduction in salt intake, and the management of stress are significant too and together they will reduce your weight and slash blood pressure.

And here is the really amazing thing:

Through my experience I am convinced that the impact of these FAT BOB SLIM actions together are far greater than simply "going on a diet." There is an added efficacy, a collective, cumulative health punch and the results they bring to bear on your high blood pressure should not be underestimated.

Scientific study notes that for every 1kg (2.2 lbs) of weight loss systolic blood pressure will reduce by 1.05 mmHg and diastolic by 0.92 mmHg.[xxvii] Yet, by 60 days of FAT BOB SLIM I had lost 28 lbs or 13kg.

Now, I was never a mathematical wizard as my son will testify but if my systolic blood pressure had fallen by 1.05 mm Hg per Kg of weight loss I would have expected a reduction of 13 × 1.05 = 13.65 mmHg yet my actual reduction was an astonishing 59 mm Hg. And my actual diastolic reduction was 21 mm Hg against an expected of 13 × 0.92 = 11.96 mm Hg.

As I said, my FAT BOB SLIM regime delivers added efficacy, a collective, cumulative punch that simply slashes high blood pressure.

Now, I'm not daft enough to believe this will work for everyone. We humans are all different. But interestingly I noted a study by Dr Michelle Harvie of 115 women who were followed over a 3 month period on a 5:2 calorie restricted diet. Dr Harvie found that on average they experienced an 11% fall in blood pressure, with some dropping by up to 38%.[xxviii]

Friend, with results like these you have to agree that FAT BOB SLIM is worth a go?

Keep with the walking.

Dump the fast food.

Get rid of the salt.

Eat 3 square meals a day and lots of vegetables too.

Fast 2 days a week.

Soon you too will slash your blood pressure. If it happened for FAT BOB SLIM it can happen for you too.

Now get ready for some yoga breathing to help you bring your blood pressure down even more...

Yoga breathing for blood pressure reduction

Stress is a killer.

The thing is it just creeps up on you bit by bit.

I know it did with me.

The change is small, imperceptibly so.

But the impact is enormous.

High blood pressure that leads to heart attack, stroke, seizure...

Stress will wear you down. It will release chemicals into the blood stream and raise your blood pressure. Not bad in a fight or flight moment but 24/7 it pushes you over the edge.

And stress is good at its job.

It celebrates in knowing it has brought down another fine man or woman.

My fellow Scotsman Jack Black, now an exceptional motivational speaker, tells how as a struggling social worker in Glasgow, fighting for his clients, working hard to make ends meet for his family, doing overtime, and organising sports outings caused him to crash out.

That is stress for you.

If you have regular headaches the chances are that's stress too.

Regular tension headaches used to be my bugbear. I was forever popping pills and drinking coffee out the office vending machine to combat its effects. But it would reappear again no matter how hard I tried to get rid of it. It was like a plague of mice: as soon as I had batted down one, another would pop its head up.

Stress should not be underestimated.

It specialises in raising your blood pressure, giving you upset stomachs, disturbing your sleep, and turning you into a depressive, negative thinking wreck.

As the growing number of people off sick from their work will testify, it is good at its job – oh the irony!

FAT BOB SLIM can look back and say that stress encouraged me to eat and drink too much. Stress was there for me when no one else was. It is devious. It is not to be trusted. The eating and drinking it introduced me to was a sort of comfort. Fatty and sugary food is like that; it gives a quick feel-good kick. But for me the kick didn't last long enough and the remedy was to turn once more to food and drink for solace – a vicious cycle if ever there was one.

Stress had fooled me into thinking it was my friend.

And then my headaches would start all over again.

And my thinking became negative.

And my heart began to race like an express train.

My palms sweated.

My mouth dried out.

I needed the toilet – too often.

If like me you have experienced any of these symptoms you too have invisibly been courted by none other than stress.

As I said: stress should not be underestimated.

This is particularly true if you are overweight and have high blood pressure.

If that is you, you need to manage your condition and get it under control quickly before stress sucks you up and spits you out with glee.

And one of the simplest things you can do to combat the ill effects of stress is to learn to breathe slowly.[xxix]

Yes, you caught me correctly: breathe slowly.

Scientific research indicates that blood pressure and anxiety are both reduced through slow breathing.

As my own blood pressure was shooting through the roof I decided to give yoga breathing a go - call me an old hippy if you want.

So what exactly is slow breathing?

The researchers noted it was 6 breaths per minute: 5 seconds of inspiration followed by 5 seconds of expiration.

Next time I sat to take my blood pressure I gave slow breathing a go. I got into the rhythm of it quickly. And it certainly made me feel calm. Better still was that the more I practised it the lower my blood pressure readings were becoming.

Could this really be true?

Or, was I just deluding myself with a fancy yoga breathing trick?

Ever the cynic that I am I didn't buy it.

I did, however, give the scientists the benefit of the doubt and decided to personally experiment with slow breathing: 15 minutes twice a day while taking my blood pressure readings.

What I experienced began to blow me away. Not at first I accept but a few weeks after starting I could see a real impact on my blood pressure readings.

It was as if I was on a different planet too.

Serenity.

But I was still convinced it was just a clever way of tricking my body. If I stopped would my blood pressure go back to its hypertensive state?

So I put it to the test.

I temporarily stopped my slow yoga breathing.

My next set of blood pressure reading were slightly higher than expected but not by much. The scientists it seems are spot on: slow breathing helps reduce stress and lowers your blood pressure too.

Now, as a scientist by training I can't conclusively conclude that slow breathing alone induced a positive downward effect on my blood pressure as I was also losing weight, eating more vegetables, reducing my salt intake and exercising at the same time. These features of the FAT BOB SLIM regime have a great impact too.

There is a collective, cumulative health punch from these activities that you simply cannot ignore or underestimate.

My advice is this: anything you can do to reduce stress and cut your blood pressure is well worth the effort.

Slow breathing helped FAT BOB SLIM.

It is also easy to do.

For me yoga breathing cut the stress of knowing I had high blood pressure. That alone was more than useful.

It helped me focus on the things that really mattered like regular exercise, eating more vegetables, reducing my salt intake, and fasting to lose weight.

Together these things began to bring my blood pressure way, way down.

The collective, cumulative health punch was at last working in my favour.

It had taken just under 2 months for my systolic blood pressure reading to be within the optimum range. It took a further month for my diastolic to similarly react.

Today, my blood pressure is well under control. I am safely within the optimum ranges for systolic and diastolic readings.

I average 100/70.

Not bad for a 50 year old man from Glasgow.

You can do it too my friend.

You can manage the stress.

You can cut your blood pressure even further.

All you have to do is breathe slowly.

Breathe in: 1,2,3,4,5; breathe out: 1,2,3,4,5.

Relax.

Know that your FAT BOB SLIM plan is working in your favour.

Keep with your daily walking.

Keep packing your plate with vegetables.

Keep the junk food at arms-length.

Keep to three square meals each day.

Keep the salt to a minimum.

Keep to your fasting schedule.

Keep relaxing.

Keep monitoring your blood pressure.

And when the downward blood pressure trend begins smile and know that your FAT BOB SLIM regime is about to deliver a major health benefit.

Everyone's a winner

When I first started my FAT BOB SLIM regime I met with immediate resistance.

My wife, God bless her, doesn't like change.

My friends openly, and with more than a touch of hostility, referred to my desire to lose weight as "nonsense!"

Those same friends just happened to be overweight.

It was as if my actions were an affront to them. Perhaps they knew deep down they too should act? Perhaps they somehow felt as if they were losing a member of the clan?

Their trusted ally FAT BOB SLIM was going AWOL!

For them they had deluded themselves into believing it was cool to be fat. It was cool to carry a protruding beer belly. It was cool to wear 40+ inch trousers. It was cool to sport outsized clothing that would be too big even for the Honey Monster to wear.

My friend, old habits die hard.

But worse than that: friends with old habits that die hard, die young.

Verily, verily I say unto you: friends with old habits that die hard, die young.

To continue my religious overtone: if it were not so, I would have told you.

My friend, FAT BOB SLIM is just a man. I am made of flesh and blood. But the medical facts before you are plain. If you don't change your unhealthy habits expect to die young.

So you have a choice to make.

And a big part of that choice will be how you react to the resistance you will inevitably encounter.

Do you commit to your FAT BOB SLIM regime or do you continue to do what you have always done?

Is the risk that you will look odd?

Is it that you will lose your friends?

Will your partner resent your personal transformation?

How can you stay strong throughout the storm?

How can you do this and make a real success of it?

I am certain these thoughts will strike you as much as they struck me at the outset of my FAT BOB SLIM journey.

My experience is that resistance is everywhere, it comes from every quarter, it is unrelenting; it is inevitable...

It will be your partner going in a huff because you don't want the usual week-end take-away. It will be your son or daughter going in a strop because you no longer buy fizzy, sugary drinks or stock the kitchen cupboards with crisps and chocolate bars. It will be your friends who now find you a kill joy because you don't want to drink excessive volumes of lager on a Saturday night out. It will be your colleagues, who despite you telling them about your commitment to FAT BOB SLIM, will offer you a wee biscuit, not just a biscuit but a "wee" biscuit, a pastry, a piece of cake or a celebratory chocolate. It will be the local hamburger restaurant that thinks a flaccid piece of lettuce and a thin slice of tomato is considered a portion of vegetables. It will be the supermarket that would rather promote a 2-for-1 offer on crisps and sugary drinks than make fruit and vegetables an inexpensive, compelling must-have for the ordinary man and woman. It will be the vending machines at the sports centres having a laugh at you: "Hey FAT BOB don't pass by without buying one of my mouth-watering sugary snacks – you know you want one, I'm here for you anytime!" It will be the TV and internet adverts for junk food or the incessant flyers for pizza through your letterbox...

With this unremitting tide of resistance and temptation it is easy to give up and return to the comfort of your old ways: old habits die hard.

But here is the really magical thing about FAT BOB SLIM: after a short spell it becomes infectious.

Seriously!

And in a good way too!

My wife, God bless her, doesn't like change. But even she soon became a convert. I swear there is something special, almost a kind of alchemy, about living the FAT BOB SLIM lifestyle. It has a special energy all of its own that transcends the ether, negates the wall of resistance, and wins over your friends and family.

As for my wife: out of the blue she announced she would be joining me on my Thursday fast day. How about that? As I said something special happens when you progress with FAT BOB SLIM. Then she decided to experiment by making a delicious low salt, vegetable-packed, minestrone soup. It was awesome! And as a lover of vegetables she is more than willing to pack her plate with broccoli, cabbage, cauliflower, peppers, red onions, tomatoes – you name it, she loves it. Together we have caught the buzz. We have become the FAT BOB SLIM team on a mission. And the really great thing is, when not at work, my wife increasingly comes out on my daily walks. But best of all is this: in just 2.5 months she has lost over 14 lbs and is looking great.

FAT BOB SLIM is infectious.

Soon others will be walking with you and not fighting against your fine ambition.

Goodness, even my Hershey-handed son, without prompting announced he had a new eating strategy: rather than consume a chocolate bar every day he would have one every second day, and rather than have a sugary drink each day he would have one only on certain days of the week – his Friday night one is a real treat, something he gets excited about, something to look forward to rather than just expecting.

And the net result for my Hershey-handed son: in the same 2.5 months he has lost a bit of a tub and over 10 lbs, taking him down safely into the healthy weight range on the BMI scale. He too joins me on my weekend walks and sleeps like a log as a result.

Note: The doctors recommend that children don't fast as they are still growing. Eating healthily and regular exercise, however, has an awesome impact on kids.

As for my friends, the ones who were so resistant to losing a trusted member of the clan, well, now they pat me on the back and say things like: "Keep up the good work Bob, you're looking great," "That walking is doing you the world of good," "That jacket fits you perfectly now," and best of all they no longer call me a "FAT BOB;" instead, they call me "SLIM BOB."

FAT BOB has become a SLIM BOB.

Some people even ask me, "What's your secret?" And I can't tell them because FAT BOB SLIM hasn't been published yet!

Or, if they haven't seen me for some time they exclaim, "Jeez! Have you LOST weight?" Quickly followed by, "You look SO much better!" I love these guys!

And the really heart-warming thing is when someone comes up to me to confess, "You've inspired me to shed weight, I so needed an incentive."

That my friend is priceless.

And it is a reminder that FAT BOB SLIM has a special energy of its own.

It is infectious.

It overcomes resistance.

It wins over the doubters.

And it inspires others to get involved.

So stay the course my friend.

Let your actions speak louder than words.

Let others marvel at your new slimline look.

Let your doctor congratulate you on slashing your blood pressure.

Let your partner join you on one or two of your fast days.

Let your friends become inspired by your achievements.

And let your new life begin...

As Errol Brown of pop group Hot Chocolate once sang, "Everyone's a winner, baby, that's the truth..."

And one last thing...

At the turn of the year I was a FAT BOB.

Today, I am a SLIM BOB.

I am FAT BOB SLIM.

I am within my healthy weight range on the BMI scale.

I have slashed my blood pressure and it is now within the optimum range and averages 100/70.

That is pretty awesome for a 50 year old man, particularly one from Glasgow.

I used to eat junk food, drink lager and do next to no exercise.

Today, I pack my dinner plate with vegetables, I drink water and herbal teas, and walk for an hour every day.

And here's the thing:

> "If a 220 lbs pizza munching, lager swilling Glaswegian can do it – so can you!"

It is so easy to sleepwalk into bad health and an early grave. But it doesn't have to be that way. The new healthy, slimline you is simply waiting to be unearthed.

And the key to that unearthing is my FAT BOB SLIM regime.

Now that you've read about it take the next step and try it out.

When it begins to work for you spread the word.

Come and join me on Twitter and Facebook.

Tell your friends about what you have done, how you lost weight, slashed your blood pressure, and feel rejuvenated.

Look out for me and, better still, come join me on one of my daily walks.

And finally, if ever I put weight back on, if ever I give up on eating vegetables, if ever I give up my daily walks, I give you permission to shout at me:

"Hey FAT BOB - SLIM!"

I'll be ever so grateful.

References————————————

[i] Dr Michael Mosley & Mimi Spencer, The Fast Diet, Short Books, 2013, pp back cover.

[ii] An urgent exercise in dealing with obesity, The Herald, 7th February 2014.

[iii] Annie Ferland, MD, MSC, Patrice Brassard, MSC, Paul Poirier, MD, PHD, FRCPC, FACC, FAHA, Is Aspartame Really Safer in Reducing the Risk of Hypoglycemia During Exercise in Patients With Type 2 Diabetes? Diabetesjournals.org, July 2007.

[iv] Michael Marra, singer/song-writer, originator of Mother Glasgow.

[v] Audrey Gillan, In Iraq, life expectancy is 67. Minutes from Glasgow city centre, it's 54, The Guardian, 21st January 2006.

[vi] Nutrition-and-you.com, Vegetable nutrition facts.

[vii] Ibid

[viii] Ibid

[ix] Ibid

[x] Rhys Blakely, Why one of the world's top cancer doctors thinks he can help you live longer, The Times Magazine, 1st March 2014, pp 20.

[xi] Matt Roberts, Fitness for life manual, Dorling Kindersley, 2011.

[xii] Ibid

[xiii] Fitnessmotivators.com

[xiv] Dr Michael Mosley & Mimi Spencer, The Fast Diet, Short Books, 2013, pp 22.

[xv] Dr Michael Mosley & Mimi Spencer, The Fast Diet, Short Books, 2013, pp 23.

[xvi] Weightlossresources.co.uk, Daily Calorie Intake.

[xvii] Dr Michael Mosley & Mimi Spencer, The Fast Diet, Short Books, 2013, pp 55.

[xviii] www.jentezenfranklin.org/types-of-fasts/

[xix] www.bloodpressureuk.org/microsites/salt/Home/Whysaltisbad

[xx] www.nhs.uk, How much salt is good for me?

[xxi] Ibid

[xxii] www.cdc.gov/features/dssodium/

[xxiii] http://dashdiet.org/low_salt_diet.asp

[xxiv] www.nhs.uk/Change4Life/Pages/healthy-eating.aspx

[xxv] Instruction Manual, OMRON, Digital Automatic Blood Pressure Monitor Model M2 Basic, pp 33.

[xxvi] US Department of Health and Human Services, Your Guide to lowering

Blood Pressure, p4.

[xxvii] Neter JE, Stam BE, Kok FJ, Grobbee DE, Geleijnse JM, Influence of weight reduction on blood pressure: a meta-analysis of randomized control trials, US National Library of Medicine, National Institutes of Health.

[xxviii] http://thefastdiet.co.uk/forums/users/clare/replies/

[xxix] Heather Mason, Matteo Vandoni, Giacomo deBarbieri, Erwan Codrons, Veena Ugargol, Luciano Bernardi, Cardiovascular and Respiratory Effect of Yogic Slow Breathing in the Yoga Beginner: What Is the Best Approach? www.hindawi.com/journals/ecam/2013/743504/

Printed in Great Britain
by Amazon.co.uk, Ltd.,
Marston Gate.